TABLE OF CONTENTS

About this book

After treating clients since 1989, in 2000, I realized my clients would benefit from documented pain management self treatment techniques. I decided to write a comprehensive book which was called *A Beginner's Guide to the Self-Treatment of Muscle Spasms*. That book grew several times and in 2008 I published *Treat Yourself to Pain Free Living*. The book has proved valuable for many readers worldwide who were suffering from chronic or acute pain and sports injuries. My clients, both at the office and on the internet, were thrilled with the ability to self-treat aches and pains that had bothered them for years.

In the case of athletes, they were grateful that they could learn how to quickly release pains that were preventing them from working out, or forcing them to drop out of a race. They appreciated that even during a race they would be able to stop, release the pain, and then keep on going.

Recognizing that many individuals have pain in one area of the body only and they don't want a book about the entire body, I decided a solution for these individuals would be to have separate books for each situation. The *Stop Pain Fast!* series was born. Each book is a small subset of the *Treat Yourself to Pain Free Living* book and provides the same valuable information and proven techniques, while focusing on just one area of the body.

You may enjoy visiting my website http://www.StopPainTheEasyWay.com and after reading the site, visiting the forum at http://forum.julstrointernational.com/ where you can read threads that may shed more light on your situation.

The Big Picture

When I went to massage school in 1988, I figured I was the only person in the class who didn't have a clue about what was happening under my skin. Wrong! I came to find out that my classmates were as much in the dark as I was. Since then I've learned that most people have a small scattering of knowledge, but they avoid the topic like the plague because they think it's too complicated. So if you are unaware of the mechanisms that move your body through space, you are in good company.

I have good news and I have bad news. First, the bad news: the body is complicated. Now, the good news: you only need a handful of information to be able to release aches and pains quickly. That bit of knowledge comes in the form of having a little body logic and learning how to read some colorful charts that become your roadmap of where to self-treat. Everything you really need to know is here in this chapter. The rest is a piece of cake.

The Frame of Our "House"

I like to think of the body as the house we live in. Like every house, we need a strong frame. We've all seen a skeleton, either on a Halloween card or at our doctor's office. The skeleton is the frame of our personal "house."

The Logic of the Body

Like computers, the body is very logical when you understand it. There is a ditty (which means a little thought or simple saying) that says, "How do you eat an elephant? One bite at a time!" That's what I'm doing here. I'm breaking down the elephant-sized mass of information and making it bite-sized for you. Plus, there's a lot that won't even make it into this book because it's not relevant to the subject of why muscles cause pain and what to do about it.

Here are 10 keys of body logic:

- Bones are just a place to attach muscles and to keep us from moving like a jellyfish.

- Muscles go in almost straight lines from a stationary point to a movable point.

- The connecting points are always on a bone.

- The muscle crosses over a joint 99% of the time.
- Muscles always pull; they never push.
- When a muscle pulls, the joint bends and you move.
- If a muscle is tight, it is pulling on the movable bone and you can't move in the opposite direction.
- When you feel pain in a joint, look for the muscle that inserts there and you'll have the source of your pain
- Pressing on these points will cause the muscle to relax and stop the tension.
- Stretching is great – when it is done properly.

That's it. You now know more about muscles than the majority of people in the world. Re-read each sentence above slowly and give it a little thought before you move on to the next sentence.

Why Muscles Cause Pain

I'm constantly hearing people say to me: "I've been doing this movement all my life. It never hurt before. I must be getting old." Baloney! You are not getting old. I use an analogy that explains exactly what is happening to your muscles.

Pretend you are a very young child standing between a bottomless well filled with water and a big rain barrel. You have an eyedropper and you are going back and forth between the well and the barrel, filling the barrel a few drops at a time. You do this for hours every day, year after year.

Every now and then you take out a glass of water or even a pot of water, but you still keep going back and forth. As you get older and you're able to stay up later in the day, you're now going back and forth for longer periods each day. Suddenly, when you're about 40 years old, your rain barrel overflows. Amazing! You tell all your friends, "I just don't understand. I've been doing this all my life and it never overflowed before." You can easily see that the problem is that you never emptied your rain barrel. It is the same with muscles.

Stick with me; this is easy to understand. Movements, especially if they are repetitive and done with strength, cause a waste byproduct called lactic acid to fill your muscles. This causes the muscle fibers to slowly shorten or even form knots in the fibers. It's a common thing for this situation to become apparent around the time you turn 40. You say, "I've been doing this all of my life. Oh, well. I must be getting old!" Do you see my point? You aren't getting old. You just never emptied out your rain barrel. This book will teach you how to how to empty your muscles of the toxins that cause the muscles to tie into knots and then how to untie the knots (spasms) in your fibers. Prevention at its best!

Lactic Acid and Other Toxins

Muscle action creates a waste product called lactic acid. The body has the ability to remove lactic acid from the muscles, but it's not at the same speed that your active body is producing it. It had been believed that excess lactic acid caused the muscles to contract into a spasm, which is also called a trigger point or a knot, putting strain on the two insertion points. However, recent research has shown that the body converts lactic acid and uses it. At this point the most recent understanding is that it is the H+ ions in lactic acid that is causing the pain and spasms. That could change in the future as science learns even more about the body

Press down on the knot and then slide deeply along the muscle to lengthen them. These two movements cause a void in the muscle fiber that the body fills with blood. The blood nourishes the fibers, and the movement stretches the fibers and releases the tension on the bones. You'll feel when the knot unties because it won't hurt the way it did before. You may even feel the knot disappear. Now is the best time to stretch.

Why the Knot in the Muscle Hurts at the Joint

It's as simple as 1-2-3.

1. A muscle merges into a fiber called a tendon.

2. The tendon inserts on a bone.

3. When the muscle pulls, the tendon gets taut and the bone moves.

Which brings me to another analogy: if you pull your hair, your head will hurt. That is exactly the way muscles can cause pain. As I just mentioned, in order for your joints to move, a muscle pulls and the bone moves. But if the muscle is tight, it is pulling even when you aren't trying to move, and it hurts. Release the tension of the muscle, and the pain goes away. A knot in the muscle always hurts to the touch. Many people believe if it's hurting, leave it alone, but the opposite is actually what you should be doing. If it hurts, work it out.

If you contract (pull) the bulk of the muscle (known as the belly of the muscle), it will hurt where the tendon of the muscle inserts into the bone. For example, when your calf muscles are contracted, they may hurt directly on the muscle. The calf muscles (gastrocnemius and soleus) merge into the Achilles tendon and insert into your heel. Since the calf muscles are pulling the tendon and it is pulling on the insertion, your heel may hurt – even when you aren't feeling anything in the calf.

Repetitive Strain Injury (RSI)

The muscles of the human body are in use 24 hours a day, 7 days a week, and 365 days a year. Despite this enormous amount of use, most of us spend little or no time caring for our muscles.

Obviously, with such extensive and continued use, we must experience "wear and tear." In medical terms this is known as repetitive strain injury, which is abbreviated as RSI. Repetitive strain injury, as the name implies, develops when a muscle is used over and over again in the same manner. Eventually the muscle fibers become strained and shortened, resulting in pain, numbness, and loss of flexibility to the areas involved. Let's face it: we are all creatures of habit. We tend to do the same things in the same way, over and over again. The way we sit, stand, walk, drive, read a book, exercise, work at a computer – and any other movement – are all important elements to the condition of our muscles.

Whether you are a homemaker or a construction worker, a typist or an interstate trucker, a musician or an electrician, the stress and strain placed on your muscles each and every day is enormous!

Repetitive strain injuries, or "wear and tear," tend to occur most often when muscles are used repeatedly. The more strength you use in the movement, the more stress is placed on the muscle. However, you do not need to be moving to be using a muscle.

While quietly sitting and reading a book, although seeming relaxed, the muscles of the fingers, hands, and arms are all in use. The same goes for the neck and low back muscles. It's ironic, isn't it, that you can be the victim of repetitive strain injury while quietly sitting in your easy chair, reading a book. In fact, sitting is a very common cause of low back pain.

Sitting for an extended period of time will cause low back pain because of a muscle named iliopsoas (pronounced "ill-ee-o-SO-as"). This muscle causes a great deal of painful problems throughout the body, from your neck to your feet.

This brings me to another phenomenon called muscle memory.

Muscle Memory

When a muscle is held in a shortened state for a period of time, it will actually shorten to become that contracted length. For example, when you move your fingers over and over, such as when you're on a computer or playing an instrument, the muscles of your forearm shorten. It's as if your body said, "Well, you're not supposed to be that short, but if that's what you want, no problem." Poof! The muscle is now short.

The problem is the muscle is still attached to the same two points on the bone, so it's pulling hard on the attachments, especially the insertion point. Since most insertion points are at a joint, you have pain in the joint. You also can't move the joint freely because of the tension the tight muscle is putting on the bone. And you can easily get an inflammation at the joint, as well as swelling caused by the fluids that build up at the site of an inflammation. These symptoms mimic arthritis.

I'm happy to say that this entire series of books are about how you can release the tension in the muscles and on the joint. Personally I find it fascinating that joint pain can frequently be self-treated so easily and quickly.

Important factors to muscle injury are:

- the amount of force exerted
- the length of time the muscle group is in use
- the angle your body is holding while you are using the muscle
- the time spent on relaxing and stretching

Sometimes it's obvious. You mowed the lawn or shoveled snow from the walk or started an aerobics class and the next day you are sore, or maybe you had low back pain the day after lifting heavy boxes. These are simple cause-and-effect injuries. However, very often it is much less obvious. A contracted muscle in the neck or chest might cause pain and discomfort to the wrist and hand, which are the symptoms of carpal tunnel syndrome, but there isn't any pain in the neck or chest. This is known as referred pain.

Okay, take a breath. You're one-third of the way through this. It's not so bad, right? If you read it slowly and visualize what is happening, it all becomes so clear. The body is wonderful. It doesn't play tricks on you. It's predictable, at least as far as muscle and joint pain is concerned.

How We Move and Other Interesting Info

As children, we used to sing a funny little song about bones. I've adapted it here because it's just perfect to begin our discussion about how we move. If you know the tune, just sing along with me.

> ♫ *The head bone's connected to the neck bone,*
>
> *and the neck bone's connected to the back bone.*
>
> ♫ *The back bone's connected to the shoulder bone*
>
> *…just see them hanging down.*

The shoulder bone's connected to the arm bone,

> ♫ *and the arm bone's connected to the wrist bones.*
>
> *The wrist bone's connected to the hand bones*

…and the fingers are there too.

> ♫ *Oh those bones, those bones,*
>
> *those skeleton bones.*

Those bones, those bones,

those skeleton bones.

Those bones, those bones,

> ♫ *those skeleton bones.*
>
> *…just see them hanging down.*

The back bone's connected to the rib bones,

and the low back affects the hip and thigh bone.

> ♫ *The thigh bone's connected to the leg bone*
>
> *…with the knee in the middle.*
>
> ♫ *The leg bone's connected to the ankle bone*
>
> *And the ankle bone's connected to the foot bone.*

The foot bone's connected to the toe bones.

… just see them hanging down!

Oh those bones, those bones,

those skeleton bones.

🎵 *Those bones, those bones,*

those skeleton bones.

Those bones, those bones,

🎵 *those skeleton bones.*

... and still nothing can move!

Adapted from "Dry Bones," author and copyright unknown.

The key words in the song are "and still nothing can move!" What makes our skeleton dance?

Muscles. Stay with me. It's pretty simple when you understand some basic concepts.

Without muscles you are like that poor skeleton – just hanging on a hook and not moving. So now we're going to get into the real meat of the subject, the "why" of a whole lot of topics, such as how muscles move your bones, some thoughts about bone spurs and tight joints, and a little bit of a lot of other interesting things.

How our Bodies are Constructed

We have 300 muscles in our bodies that are duplicated on each side, giving us a total of 600 muscles. Now, aren't you glad I said it isn't important for you to learn the names and actions of each muscle, and don't you have a lot more respect for your local massage therapist who does know them?

How a Muscle Moves a Joint

Muscles are just pulleys that are attached to a bone on both ends. A muscle crossing over a joint gives that joint the ability to move. As mentioned above, movement of a joint is a two-step process: one muscle must contract and shorten while the opposing muscle must relax and lengthen. When a knot occurs in the muscle, it will shorten the fibers. The pain is usually felt at the insertion of the muscle (the place where the muscle tendon attaches to the bone), which is at the joint.

In my office I'm constantly explaining the body to my clients by using simple comparisons. In this case we will compare the way a muscle moves a bone by comparing it to the way an electric motor opens a garage door.

Each muscle or muscle group has its own unique function. Some muscles work alone; however, most muscles work together as a team. When one muscle is pulling, the opposite muscle is stretching. Then to reverse the movement, the muscles change roles and the stretched muscle will pull while the shortened muscle will stretch. When the muscle that is supposed to stretch is tight, it will prevent you from moving in that direction. It sounds a bit confusing until you think through the explanation I always use at my office:

When you open your garage door with an electric motor, you

1. Send the message with a "clicker" to turn on the motor.

2. The motor pulls on a cable that lifts your garage door.

3. The door opens and stays that way until the motor releases the tension and lets the cable lengthen and then the door comes down.

In our example, the "clicker" is the nerve impulse sending a message to the muscle, the motor is the muscle, the cable is the tendon that crosses over a joint to insert into a bone, and in this case the bone is the bottom of the garage door.

As a muscle "turns on" (or shortens), the tendon pulls on the bone where it is attached. Since this bone is on the other side of a joint, the joint bends. When the muscle releases the tension, the tendon stops pulling. Now the muscle that moves the bone in the opposite direction can work and pull the bone so it moves back to where it was originally by pulling it in the other direction.

You can imagine that if the contracted muscle doesn't release all the way, the bone can't go back to its original position, and if you try to move it, it will hurt.

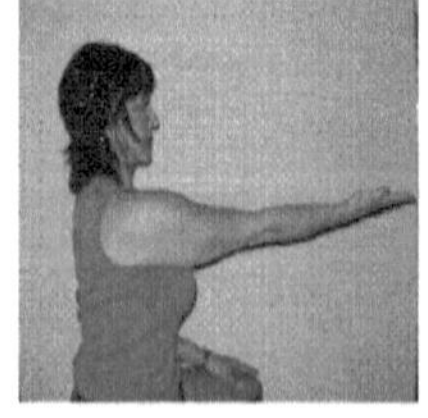

This is easy to explain by using your elbow for a demonstration and watching what happens when you go to touch your shoulder. An important piece to this is the fact that both the biceps and the triceps cross over your elbow joint and insert on the bone of your lower arm. In both cases, a tight muscle will strain your elbow joint. A tight biceps will hurt the inside of your elbow, and a tight triceps will hurt the outside of your elbow.

When your arm is straight, your triceps muscle is contracted to its shortest length and your biceps muscle is fully stretched. If your biceps muscle is tight, you won't be able to put your arm out all the way.

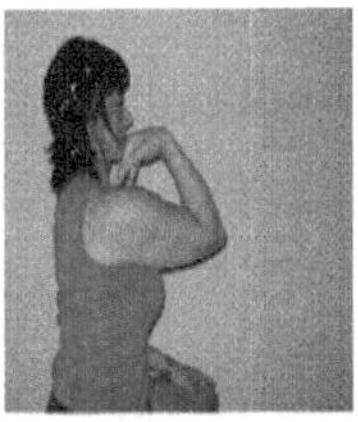

In order for you to touch your shoulder, your biceps will contract, but the triceps on the back of your upper arm must stretch. If your triceps muscle is tight, you'll only be able to go as far as the triceps will stretch and then you'll stop.

If you can't touch your shoulder without pain to your elbow, many therapists will tell you that you need to strengthen your biceps, but they aren't even considering that your triceps are tight and won't let your arm bend. If you release the tension on the triceps, you can bend your arm just fine. It's simple logic, but then the body is incredibly logical when we listen to it.

Every movement the body makes uses this same principle. One muscle shortens to cause the movement and another muscle lengthens to allow the movement. This other muscle is called the opposing muscle because it is doing the opposite movement, so the biceps muscle opposes the triceps muscle and the triceps opposes the biceps.

Knots, Trigger Points, Joint Pain, and Stretching

As you just read, when a muscle pulls, a bone moves. Now let's talk about what happens when a knot forms in a muscle. To recap, a muscle originates on a stationary bone and then inserts into a movable bone.

Let's change those bones to trees…

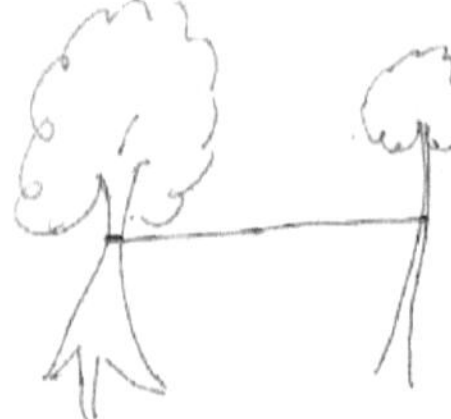

In this analogy the stationary bone is a big solid tree, the muscle is a rope, and the movable bone is a slender flexible tree. When the rope has just the right tension, it will be straight across the middle and the flexible tree will be standing up.

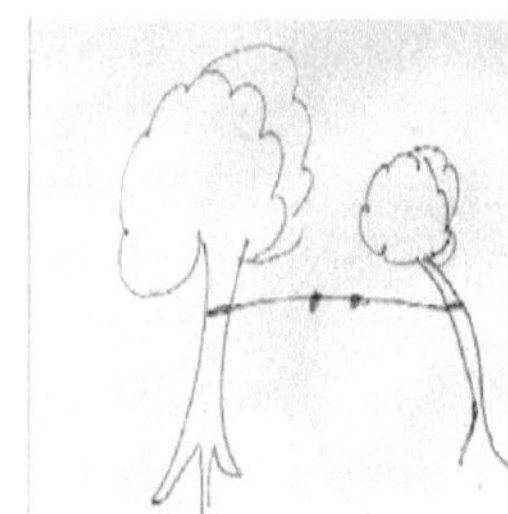

When a knot is tied in the rope, the flexible tree will bend, and if several knots are tied in the rope, the tree is really bent over. You can see that the flexible tree won't stand up straight again until the knots are untied.

In the same way, a knot in your muscle fibers will pull on the movable bone and you won't be able to move properly without putting a great deal of strain on the movable bone.

If you try to push the flexible tree up straight without first untying the knots, you can imagine that you'll be making the knots tighter, overstretching the rest of the rope, and the fibers may even tear.

These knots are actually spasms, which are also called trigger points. The trigger points are all over your body and would be a huge challenge to locate if not for the work of two medical doctors, Janet Travell and David Simons. Drs Travell and Simons proved that trigger points all over the body will refer pain and numbness to areas that are often far from the spasm. Their landmark research was documented in a two books titled *Myofascial Pain and Dysfunction, The Trigger Point Manual*. These books were key to my work and I've taken their research and put it onto user-friendly charts to help you see where to find the trigger points and where each point will refer pain and/or numbness. To view the Trigger Point charts for the entire body you can go to <u>www.charts.julstro.com/index.html</u>

Why Stretching May Hurt

If you try to stretch a muscle that is tied up in knots, you will make the trigger point more complex and you'll overstretch the muscle fibers on either side of the knot. In fact, you could feel worse after stretching than you did before.

The Julstro™ techniques show you how to do twofold stretches by pressing on a trigger point while stretching at the same time. And, of course, just releasing the knot first and then doing some regular stretches will work just fine. Each *Stop Pain FAST!* book demonstrates how to do one or two of the Julstro™ treatments and stretches that are applicable to that books topic.

The charts will be helpful as you read each book.

A Charley Horse or Cramp

A muscle is actually a big bundle of thousands or millions of individual fibers. Inside the muscle are smaller and smaller bundles of muscles, each covered with a strong cover called myofascia that just holds the fibers in place. Each fiber pulls independently, with more fibers being used in order to do movements that require more strength.

Each individual muscle fiber operates according to the "all or nothing" principle. This means that when the muscle fiber is stimulated, it will contract with all its force. It will not stop in the middle of the contraction. There is no middle of the road with a muscle. It is all or nothing.

In reality, and under certain adverse conditions, all the fibers in a muscle might suddenly contract and remain "stuck" in the contracted position. This causes an acute pain, such as a cramp (commonly called a charley horse), which can be severe.

Usually, however, the results of shortened muscle fibers occur slowly and are more subtle. The resulting "knot" is actually a spasm which pulls on both ends of the muscle with more force placed on the insertion point of the muscle at the joint. For example, shortened muscles might be the cause of someone's "hunchback," chronic headache, or carpal tunnel syndrome.

Power depends on how many fibers are contracting, which is why you can use the same group of muscles to pick up a feather or a heavy weight. In the normal course of events you unconsciously control the number of fibers being used and the speed of the contraction.

A charley horse, or cramp, is a shocking (to put it mildly) break from the norm. All of a sudden every fiber in a muscle shortens totally with such force that you feel like you've been hit by a moving train. You either sit bolt upright in bed (if you were sleeping) or end up in a heap on the floor (if you were standing), and panic immediately sets in as your muscle screams for attention.

You sure don't want to be looking for this book if you ever get a cramp. You want to immediately know how to do the treatments. Usually this happens in your calf, although it sometimes happens to your hamstrings in the back of your thigh, or in your foot. I've put the treatments in the appropriate sections, but let's talk about some basics here.

How to Stop a Cramp

Realizing that a muscle won't stop contracting in the middle of a cramp, you need to help the fibers contract as quickly as possible. To stop the cramp you'll need to help the muscle shorten even quicker than it is, and you do this by pushing the two ends of the muscle together. Grab the muscle on either end (see each chapter for details) and push the ends together as hard as you can. Your natural tendency is to try to stretch, but don't do that – yet. Stretching while the muscle is violently contracting will cause the fibers to tear, and you'll feel pain for days or even longer. First, you need to stop the cramping motion. Then you can stretch.

Pushing the fibers together will hurt like crazy and cause you to lose your breath, but it will only be for about five of the longest seconds you've ever lived. Not pushing the muscle together will mean the cramp will take longer to complete, and you can be sure that it will complete the contraction.

After you can breathe again, continue holding the muscle together for about 60 seconds. The pain will be going down now, and you can do some deep breathing to get some oxygen into the muscles. Then just let go and continue with some more deep breaths. Do the movement for a second time, but don't worry – this time won't hurt. You just want to make sure to help any last fibers that may not have finished the contraction the first time. Once you've done the second squeeze, then you can start to push the toxins out of the fibers and draw in some blood.

Begin to knead the muscle, just like it was bread dough. Squeeze from the top of the muscle down toward the insertion. This will feel really good, so you can do it for as long as you want – the more the better. When you stop this last piece of the treatment, now it's safe to stretch the muscle.

Spasms, Trigger Points and Knots

The difference in the size and feel of contracted muscles can be caused by the number of fibers involved or, in some cases, whether the fiber is injured or just shortened by repetitive use. An explanation of the terms used to describe these conditions is interesting, although not required in order to do the Julstro™ treatments.

Spasms - Trigger Points – Knots: All three of these words mean the same thing. A spasm, or trigger point, is a knot of muscle fibers that feels like a hard bump in the muscle. It can range from small (the size of a frozen pea) to rather large (the size of your fist), but it will always feel like a knot surrounded by normal muscle fibers. As mentioned before, knots are formed by a toxic waste product of muscle action. Since our body can't flush away all the toxins that are produced during exercise or other repetitive movements, the excess lactic acid triggers the muscle fibers to shorten into a knot. The knot usually forms slowly, so most people aren't aware that they even have a spasm. As the fibers shorten into the knot, people just adjust to the discomfort and don't focus on the knot of muscle fibers.

Contractions: A contraction is a shortening of the full length of one or more muscle fibers and, depending on size or location, it either feels like a thick rope within the muscle or the entire muscle may feel thick and hard. To visualize a contraction, think of taking the muscle and pushing the two ends into the center, making the muscle shorter and thicker. The problem is that in our bodies each of the two ends of the muscle are still connected to a bone and the shortening causes a great deal of tension on the bones. In fact, if the muscle contracts too much, it will actually tear from the bone. This is often the situation when a person has an Achilles tendon tear at the heel of the foot, a rotator cuff tear, shin splints, or a torn hamstring.

You will find that each time you do the movements it will hurt less. This is because the lactic acid is being pushed out of the muscle. The knots and contractions are lengthening, and the tension is being released from the muscle fibers.

Adhesions: Adhesions feel like tight strings that aren't usually painful. In fact, you rarely know they are there. Eventually you will begin to realize that you don't have the power that you once had, and you don't know why. An adhesion is the body's way to protect an injured muscle fiber, and it is actually a phenomenon called splinting. If a fiber gets injured, it puts out a sticky substance that causes the fibers next to the injured fiber to stick to it, allowing the injured fiber to relax because it is being carried along with the adjoining fibers. This reduces the power of your muscle by taking some of the fibers out of action. Instead of each fiber working independently, giving you the ability to use all the fibers required to do the task you want, the center fibers are not working at all, decreasing your strength. As you are doing the Julstro™ techniques taught in the *Stop Pain Fast!* Series or the *Treat Yourself To Pain Free Living*, you will be releasing the bond that is holding the fibers together, thereby freeing the muscle to work efficiently.

Having worked with thousands of clients, I have found that in many cases muscles are overlooked when physicians are diagnosing painful joint problems. This is particularly true of carpal tunnel syndrome and low back pain. The muscles in these areas are rarely even considered before surgery is planned. I believe it behooves everyone prior to having surgery on any joint, including back surgery, to first check the muscles that are affecting the joint. You can read about the muscles that cause the symptoms of carpal tunnel syndrome by going to http://CarpalTunnelResults.com.

Bone Bruise

A bone bruise is extremely painful and can take months to heal. It can happen anywhere in the body and usually is caused by direct pressure on the bone, such as when a person has a fall, bangs into the bone, or pounds on the feet while running or jumping. It feels like the bone is cracked, and therefore it is wise to have it x-rayed to rule out that possibility. If the x-ray is clear, you can be sure that you are only dealing with a bruise. The pain can still be severe and can last for up to a year.

Check each of the muscles that either cross over the bruised area or insert near it so you can work at releasing the tension that is likely to be complicating the issue. For example, a bone bruise on the heel needs to have the muscles of the lower leg and foot deeply massaged so they aren't pulling on the bones of the foot. It's a catch-22 situation because the bone bruise will cause the muscles to go into a knot, and the tight muscles will negatively affect the bruised area. When possible, cushion the area from repeated shock. In the case of a bruised bone in your foot, look for thick gel pads at your local drug store. You won't be able to run on a bone bruise, and even just walking or standing will cause pain. The gel pads in your shoes will ease the pain and prevent further bruising.

Because it will be painful to put any pressure on the bruised bone, you change the way you stand or walk, and you may then cause other muscles to contract or knot. For example, in the case of a left heel bone bruise, your left leg needs to be treated all the way from your low back to your lower leg muscles. The muscles of the arch need to be treated as well. You may find you are having pain in your right low back, hip, and/or right knee. If this is the case, I suggest you work on both sides of your body, not just the side with the bone bruise. All of the muscles affecting each area need to be treated individually and frequently. They will continue to get tight for as long as the bone bruise is active, so you need to continue to release the tension. That is one of the benefits of knowing how to treat yourself – you can do it many times a day instead of just when you can get to a therapist.

An analgesic gel such as Sombra™ is great for easing muscle tension, and arnica may help lessen the muscle pain. You should speak to your doctor if you feel you need medication for swelling

Don't despair. It's definitely a challenge that seems to go on and on, but it will eventually heal.

Tendonitis: The term "tendonitis" simply means an inflammation ("itis") where the tendon attaches to the bone. It is a description, even though it is usually given as a diagnosis. However, the diagnosis doesn't give the reason for the inflammation. It just says that there is an inflammation. My years of working with clients who have been diagnosed with tendonitis have shown me that the most common cause of the inflammation is the muscle pulling so hard on the tendon that it is actually trying to tear the tendon from the bone.

To take an anti-inflammatory drug while the muscle is still in spasm is counterproductive. It's like pulling your hair and taking an aspirin for the headache. You won't get rid of the headache until you stop pulling your hair. Likewise, you won't get rid of tendonitis until you release the tension in the muscle, thereby releasing the tension where the tendon merges into the bone.

It's so logical.

When I explain to clients that we need to stop treating the symptom – the pain in the bone – and treat the muscle that is in spasm, it makes sense to them. Everything that is taught in each of the Julstro™ treatment books and DVDs focus on treating the muscles that cause tendonitis. The Julstro self-treatments are quite successful at making the inflammation go away.

Overshadowed Pain

When I was a child, if I complained to my mother about a pain she would say, "Come here and I'll step on your foot. Then you won't feel the pain." She didn't realize it at the time, but she was demonstrating overshadowed pain.

Fortunately, the brain focuses on the greatest pain, blocking out most other pains from our awareness. If this weren't the case, we'd spend all of our time focusing on the aches in our body.

When the greatest pain is eliminated, the next greatest pain appears. It is commonplace in my office to hear someone saying, "My hip feels fine, but now my shoulder hurts" (or some variation of that statement), and it's all because of overshadowed pain.

Don't be surprised if you successfully eliminate one pain and a new pain pops up. Just keep moving along and treating each pain with the techniques that are taught in this series of books, or in my full book, *Treat Yourself to Pain-Free Living*. You have the tools necessary to rid yourself of pain as it appears. Life is busy, and we all do repetitive movements so frequently that pain is inevitable, but it doesn't need to limit your life.

Bone Spurs

Another phenomenon attests to the wisdom of the body. As the muscle is pulling the tendon away from the bone, the body sends bone cells to secure the attachment. As these bone cells collect, you get what is called a spur, or a bump of bone. This is frequently seen at the heel and at the shoulder, but it can also be in your fingers, wrist, or any other joint.

In fact, in Book *#13 – Stop Trigger Finger, Wrist & Hand Pain FAST!* - as you read the section titled *A Very Special Muscle Group*, you'll read about a man who was suffering from a bone spur in his neck for nine years, causing severe head and neck pain. To try to break down the spur without first releasing the muscle tightness is fruitless. The body's intelligence will simply send more bone cells to secure the tendon.

I have worked with many people, both in my office and on my forum, who have suffered for years from bone spurs. It is wonderful to hear them report that releasing the tension in the muscles has eliminated the pain at the spur.

Numbness and Tingling

In general, pain is caused by a tight muscle pulling on its insertion point at the bone, while numbness and/or tingling are caused by pressure along a nerve anywhere from the beginning to the end of the fiber.

A muscle functions because a message is sent to it via a nerve. However, when a nerve is impinged, which means "pressed upon," either by a tight muscle or pressure from a bone, the message is interfered. The incomplete signal will cause the muscle to not react as expected, similar to static you hear on your radio when the dial is off by just a bit. In most cases when the nerve is impinged you will feel tingling or numbness, but since the muscle isn't receiving a strong contract message, you can also feel weak. If the message is broken, such as when a nerve is severed, the muscle is unable to contract at all and eventually atrophy breaks down the otherwise healthy muscle fibers.

There is a phenomenon called the phantom limb that explains why a person feels pain in a limb that has been amputated. The phantom limb theory explains why a person feels pain, tingling, or numbness at the end point when a nerve is impinged or damaged anywhere along its length. While this is happening with all nerves, the two major nerves that will cause multiple problems when pressure is applied are the brachial plexus in the neck and the sciatic nerve at the base of the spine. Also, the femoral nerve, which lies within the pelvis, will cause the front of your thigh to go numb.

A trigger point pressing into a muscle of the neck will cause numbness in the thumb and two fingers (symptoms of carpal tunnel syndrome), and pressure on the sciatic nerve will cause pain all around your hip area, as well as tingling in your hamstrings and calf and numbness in your feet. An impingement on either of these nerves will also cause weakness, pain, and tingling in other areas far from the source of the pressure.

Sprains, Broken Bones And Muscles

As a child, did you ever play with a Slinky®? This classic spring toy demonstrates what happens to a muscle when it is either overstretched from a sprain or totally contracts due to a broken bone.

The Effect of Sprains on Muscles

If you hold the Slinky® all the way out to its longest length and then suddenly just let go, the spring won't smoothly go back to its previous coil. Instead, it's going to become a big knot in the middle. The same thing happens to your muscles when they are sprained.

When you sprain a joint – for example, your ankle – the muscles of the lower leg are suddenly overstretched and then quickly released, causing multiple trigger point knots to form in each of the muscles. Since a muscle is normally held in perfect tension from the origination to the insertion, these knots will cause a stress to be placed on the insertion point of the muscle at the joint, causing pain that will not stop until the trigger points are released. As a result, you may feel pain in your ankle for years after a sprain. However, the pain will quickly go away once the knots are untied and the tension is released.

A sprain at any joint requires treatment of the knots found in each muscle that crosses that joint.

While stretching when the spasms are still shortening the muscles can cause further pain, or at best give short-lived temporary relief, stretching after the knots are treated will relieve the tension on the joint.

The Effect of Broken Bones on Muscles

Think about having an elastic band stretched from one bone to another, crossing a joint. The bone is holding the band in perfect tension. If the bone breaks, the elastic band will snap together, pulling the pieces of bone with it.

This analogy is exactly what happens to your muscles when a bone breaks and the muscle suddenly contracts totally. As the bone is set in a cast, the muscle is pulled back into place, but rarely are the tight fibers of the muscle treated to bring them back to their correct length.

This results in the bone being strained by the multiple knots that have formed in the muscle during the sudden contraction. I have seen clients who have experienced pain for years after a fracture, even though the bone has healed perfectly. As soon as the muscle spasms are treated, the pressure is removed from the bone and pain is eliminated.

Also, if you currently still have on a cast while the bone is healing, putting direct pressure onto the muscles that are just above the top of the cast will help release the tight muscles that are causing tension at the break.

The Big Question - Deciding Which to Use, a Hot or Cold Compress

Everyone gets confused about it, and there really isn't a hard-and-fast rule. I've always worked with two rules. The first rule: If the injury is less than 24 hours old or if there is swelling, use ice; if it's more than 24 hours old, use heat. If the pain is really stubborn, do a system called contrast bathing, which alternates between 10 minutes of hot and 10 minutes of cold.

The second rule: Try ice, then try heat, and see which feels better.

You Can Treat the Pain!

I have found that people are nervous about putting pressure on a painful point, usually because they believe they are causing problems rather than helping to heal the situation. I always tell people to use enough pressure that it "hurts so good" but never so much that the area "screams" in pain. I've found that once a person understands that concept, they are very good at finding the correct level of pressure to properly treat their own muscles.

The bottom line is **YOU ARE YOUR OWN BEST THERAPIST!**

Other Books and Instructional DVDs by Julie Donnelly

DVDs:

The Julstro System for Carpal Tunnel Syndrome—Hand/Wrist Pain and Numbness

The Julstro Self-Treatment Series:

Treat Your Upper Body FAST!
Treat Your Low Back FAST!
Treat Your Lower Body FAST!

Books:

Carpal Tunnel Syndrome – What You Don't Know CAN Hurt You!
The Pain-Free Athlete (coming soon)
The Pain-Free Triathlete (out of print)

The Pain-Free Runner

The Pain-Free Swimmer (out of print)
Treat Yourself to Pain-Free Living

The Secret to Your Best Golf Game Ever! (coming soon)

The Stop Pain FAST! series:

#1 – Stop Pain FAST! Discover the Secret of Why Muscles Cause Pain.

#2 – Stop Stiff Neck Pain FAST!

#3 – Stop Tension Headache Pain FAST!

#4 – Stop TMJ Pain FAST!

#5 – Stop Ear Pain and Tinnitus FAST!

#6 – Stop Whiplash Pain FAST!

#15 – Stop Low Back Pain FAST!

#16 – Stop Hip (Labral Tear) Pain FAST!

#17 – Stop Sciatica Pain FAST!

#22 – Stop Calf Cramp Pain FAST!

#24 – Stop Shin Splint Pain FAST!

#26 – Stop Plantar Fasciitis and Morton's Neuroma Pain FAST!